4 Weeks

Of Diet Menus

Easy Weight Loss

Minimal Cooking and Diet Tips

Written by
M. Funke

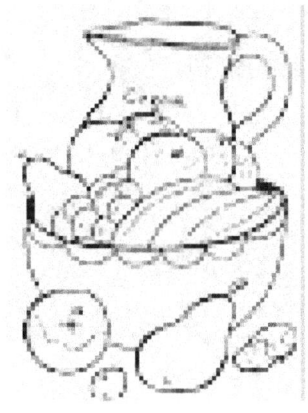

1

My Mantra

"Buy Healthy, Cook Healthy, Eat Healthy"

Contents

First Week

Second Week

Third Week

Fourth Week

Bonus Week

Introduction

This book contains breakfast meals that are easy to prepare. The choices are already made for you. Saves you time by not having to decide what to make.

Lunches are also spelled out for you. They can be eaten at home or taken with you to work. No cooking needed.

Mid-afternoon snack consists of fresh fruit. The choice is yours depending on what is in season and what you like to eat.

Dinner meals need a minimal time to prepare and cook. The menus consist of a protein such as chicken and either frozen or fresh vegetables and a salad.

Be sure to consult with your doctor before using these menus or any other.

If you make changes in the menus it will not work as well. If you replace the pita bread at lunch for two slices of bread, you are adding an additional 200 calories each day. Add that by 5 days and you have added an additional 1000 calories for the week. At the end of the four weeks that means an additional 4000 calories you do not need.

A lot of the staples bought in week one will last for the entire month.

Weigh yourself in the morning before you begin this diet and then once a week. It might be a good idea to take your measurements also, such as chest, waist, hips and thighs. Then weigh yourself once a week and again at the end of the 4 Weeks. I'll post reminders on those days for you.

Negative calorie foods are most fruits and vegetables. That means you can eat more of those and still lose weight.

Wishing you great success in your weight loss.

First Week

Weigh yourself first thing in the morning and take your measurements, chest, waist, hips and thighs.

Day 1

Breakfast	Oatmeal Weight Control 1 cup Green Tea or Coffee
	Oatmeal made with water NO MILK OR SUGAR
Lunch	3-4 oz. Sardines Pita Bread – ½ Tossed Salad with 1 tbsp. Dressing 1 cup Green Tea
	Microwave the bread for 10 seconds for ease of opening Mix the Sardines with 1-cup salad and stuff into the Pita bread
Snack	Fresh Fruit Around 3 PM
Dinner	4 oz. Flounder Red Beets – ½ small can Tossed Salad with 1 tbsp. Dressing 8 oz. Milk
	Grill or broil Flounder without breading

Add 1 tbsp. Apple Cider Vinegar to liquid in beets and let sit for about 5 minutes.

Salad Dressing

Use one packet of salad dressing – In the cruet, fill with vinegar up to the mark, add the seasoning and shake. Switch the oil and water quantities. Then in the area for water, replace with oil and fill the oil portion of the cruet with water. This does not change the taste of the dressing but eliminates most of the calories.

Day 2

Breakfast	4 Pancakes – 4-inch size 1 tsp. Jelly 1 cup Green Tea or Coffee NO MILK OR SUGAR IN DRINK Can freeze extra pancakes
Lunch	4 oz. Salmon Tossed Salad with 1 tbsp. Dressing Pita Bread – ½ 1 cup Green Tea
Snack	Fresh Fruit Around 3 PM
Dinner	4 oz. Chicken Breast 1 cup Broccoli Mixed Salad 8 oz. Milk

Grill, broil or bake the chicken. If you do all the chicken breasts at once, wrap the extras and place in a freezer bag and freeze for future meals.

Fish:

Eat fish at least seven times per week. Broil, grill or bake the fish without breading. Canned fish is quick and easy to prepare. Beware of the too fatty fish.

Cocktail Sauce:

Make your own Cocktail Sauce by adding Horseradish to ketchup. Amount depends on how hot you like it.

Day 3

Breakfast   Oatmeal Weight Control
Applesauce – Sugar Free
1 cup Green Tea or Coffee

Mix some of the Applesauce into your oatmeal, if you want

Lunch   3–4 oz. Sardines
Pita Bread – ½
Tossed Salad with 1 tbsp. Dressing
1 cup Green Tea

Snack   Fresh Fruit   Around 3 PM

Dinner   Calves Liver
½ can Red Beets
1 Onion sautéed
8 oz. Milk

Salad Ingredients:

You can use any of the fresh vegetables that you like, such as lettuce (Romaine is a good choice), shredded carrots and cabbage, cucumbers or others of your favorites in season. Sliced tomatoes are a good selection for topping sandwiches.

Day 4

Breakfast	Grapenuts – ½ cup
	Milk – ½ cup
	1 cup Green Tea or Coffee

Lunch	4 oz. Tuna
	Tossed Salad with 1 tbsp. Dressing
	Pita Bread – ½
	1 cup Green Tea

Snack	Fresh Fruit	Around 3 PM

Dinner	TV Dinner – Healthy Choice or Lean Cuisine
	Mixed Salad
	8 oz, Milk

Hate Exercise:

If you are like me, you hate exercise. But some exercise is good for you. The easiest and cheapest is walking. Don't have time to go for a walk in the park? No problem. Wear a pedometer to track the number of steps you take in a day.

One way to increase your steps is to walk up and down all the aisles in the supermarket when you go shopping. Just don't buy anything that is not on your shopping list.

Another way that is often mentioned is to park your car further from the front door of your office or place of business. I don't like this one because it could be raining when you leave work even though the sun was shining when you arrived in the morning.

Many people have mentioned walking in the enclosed malls as a way to increase exercise. This is good if you go before the stores open so you're not tempted to stop and shop. It is also great in the winter when the weather is cold outside or snowy.

Day 5

Breakfast	Eggs – 2
	Turkey Bacon – 2 slices
	1 cup Green Tea or Coffee
	Eggs cooked any way you like them
	NO SALT – just pepper or other spices
Lunch	Shrimp – 8–10 large
	Cocktail Sauce (Homemade)
	Tossed Salad
	Toast – 1 slice
	1 cup Green Tea

Snack   Fresh Fruit   Around 3 PM

Dinner	TV Dinner
	Mixed Salad
	1 cup Green Tea

Shrimp

If you buy the frozen shrimp, just take out the amount you need and return the rest to the freezer. Serve in a cocktail glass and serve with a homemade cocktail sauce, which has less salt and sugar then the store bought ones.

Day 6

Breakfast	Cottage Cheese – 4 oz. Banana – ½ Strawberries – 8 or 10 Milk – ½ cup Dash of Extract – Vanilla or Almond

Slice fruit and place all ingredients in a blender and blend until smooth.

Lunch	1 cup Lentil Soup Raisin Bread – 1 slice 1 cup Green Tea

Raisin Bread – wrap each slice individually and place in a freezer bag and freeze. Then thaw each slice, as you need it at room temperature for about 1 hour.

Snack	Fresh Fruit	Around 3 PM

Dinner	TV Dinner Mixed Salad 1 cup Green Tea

Meats:

If using meats in this diet, be sure they are lean with all fat removed. Broil, bake or grill any meat you are using. BBQ sauces are allowed.

Day 7

Breakfast	Eggs – 2
	Turkey Bacon – 2 slices
	Raisin Bread – 1 slice
	8 oz. Milk
Lunch	4 oz. Tuna
	Tossed Salad with 1 tbsp. Dressing
	Pita Bread – ½
	1 cup Green Tea
Snack	Fresh Fruit Around 3 PM
Dinner	Crab meat – Imitation – 1 cup with 1 tbsp Mayo
	7 spears Asparagus – cooked
	Mixed Salad with 1 tbsp. Dressing
	8 oz. Milk

BMI

BMI – Metabolic and weight loss calculator

When was the last time you took your BMI? (Body Mass Index)

Go to this or any website to check your BMI.

http://health.msn.com/weight-loss/bmi-calculator.aspx

Then near the end of the "4 Week Menus" I will remind you again to check your BMI to see what progress you made.

Second Week

Weigh yourself first thing in the morning and take your measurements, chest, waist, hips and thighs.

Day 8

Breakfast	4 Pancakes – 4-inch size 1 tsp. Jelly 1 cup Green Tea or Coffee NO MILK OR SUGAR IN DRINK
Lunch	3 or 4 Sardines Pita bread – ½ Tossed Salad with 1 tbsp. Dressing 1 cup Green Tea
Snack	Fresh Fruit About 3 PM
Dinner	4 oz. Chicken Breast 1 cup Broccoli Mixed Salad 8 oz Milk

Sandwiches

Prepare chicken, tuna and others with fat-free Mayonnaise

Day 9

Breakfast   Oatmeal Weight Control
1 cup Green Tea or Coffee

Lunch   4 oz. Salmon
Tossed Salad with 1 tbsp. Dressing
Pita Bread – ½
1 cup Green Tea

Snack   Fresh Fruit   Around 3 PM

Dinner   4 oz. Flounder – NO BREADING
Red Beets – ½ small can
Tossed Salad with 1 tbsp. Dressing
8 oz. Milk

Add 1 tbsp. Apple Cider Vinegar to the juice in the red beets

Natural Fat Burning Properties

Such as cayenne, ginger, green tea, cinnamon, lemon, hot peppers, and apple cider vinegar. Try to use one or two of these each day to assist in weight loss.

Day 10

Breakfast	Grapenuts – ½ cup
	½ cup Milk
	1 cup Green Tea or Coffee

Lunch   4 oz. Tuna
Tossed Salad with 1 tbsp. Dressing
Pita Bread – ½
1 cup Green Tea

Snack   Fresh Fruit   Around 3 PM

Dinner   TV Dinner
Broccoli – 1 cup
Mixed Salad
1 cup Green Tea

TV Dinner – Lean Cuisine, Healthy Choice, etc.

Spaghetti Sauce

Instead of meat in sauce, use fresh Zucchini, Mushrooms, Onions and Green Peppers.

Day 11

Breakfast	Eggs – 2	
	Turkey Bacon – 2 slices	
	1 cup Green Tea or Coffee	
Lunch	3–4 oz. Sardines	
	Pita Bread – ½	
	Tossed Salad with 1 tbsp. Dressing	
	1 cup Green Tea	
Snack	Fresh Fruit	Around 3 PM
Dinner	Crab – Imitation – ½ cup	
	1 tbsp. Mayo	
	Mixed Salad	
	Asparagus – 7 spears, cooked	
	8 oz. Milk	

Lifestyle Change

Make this a lifestyle change, not a diet. This way, you are not on a diet, so you can't fall off the diet. It takes 21 days for a habit to form and stick for life.

Day 12

Breakfast	Oatmeal Weight Control
	Apple Sauce – Sugar Free
	1 cup Green Tea or Coffee
Lunch	Shrimp – 8 large
	Homemade Cocktail Sauce for dipping
	Tossed Salad
	1 slice Bread
	1 cup Green Tea
Snack	Fresh Fruit Around 3 PM
Dinner	Healthy Choice with dessert
	Mixed Salad
	1 cup Green Tea

Soda

Ditch the sodas permanently. They contain too many empty calories.

Day 13

Breakfast   Cottage Cheese – 4 oz.
Banana – ½
Blueberries – ½ cup
Milk – ¾ cup
Dash of Extract – Vanilla or Almond

Place sliced fruit and all ingredients in a blender and blend until smooth.

Lunch   3-4 oz. Sardines
Pita Bread – ½
Tossed Salad with 1 tbsp. Dressing
1 cup Green Tea

Snack   Fresh Fruit   Around 3 PM

Dinner   Chopped Meat – ¼ lb. – 93% Lean
Whole Wheat Bread – 1 slice
Cheese, Velveeta – 1 slice
Tomato – 1 slice
Lettuce – 1 leaf

Shape meat into a patty and broil. Place cooked patty on bread and top with tomato and then slice of cheese. Broil until the cheese melts. Use the lettuce leaf as a top to the sandwich.

Clean Up Your Act

Get rid of all the junk food in your refrigerator, freezer and pantry. If it's not on hand or in the house, you can't eat it.

Day 14

Breakfast	Eggs – 2
	Turkey Bacon – 2 slices
	Raisin Bread – 1 slice
	8 oz. Milk

Lunch	1 cup Lentil Soup
	Raisin Bread – 1 slice
	1 cup Green Tea

Snack	Fresh Fruit	Around 3 PM

Dinner	Ham – 3 slices
	Crushed Pineapple – ¼ cup
	Shredded Low-fat Cheese – ¼ cup
	Whole Wheat Bread – 2 slices

Cut the ham into small pieces; mix with the pineapple and cheese, adding 1 tbsp. Mayo and spread on one slice of bread. Place second piece of bread on top and cook in a Panini pan or in a non-stick skillet. If doing on the stovetop, turn sandwich over and brown other side.

Mini Goals

Set mini goals to keep you motivated. Such as, every five pounds or every inch off your waist. Reward yourself with a small trinket or treat. Start a sort of Charm Bracelet for every ten pounds you lose.

Third Week

Weigh yourself first thing in the morning and take your measurements, chest, waist, hips and thighs.

Day 15

Breakfast   4 Pancakes – 4-inch size
                     1 tsp. Jelly
                     1 cup Green Tea or Coffee
                     NO MILK OR SUGAR IN DRINK

Lunch   3–4 oz. Sardines
                     Pita Bread – ½
                     Tossed Salad with 1 tbsp. Dressing
                     1 cup Green Tea

Snack   Fresh Fruit   Around 3 PM

Dinner   Bread Pudding:
                     2 slices Raisin Bread
                     1 Egg
                     ¼ cup Milk
                     Dash Vanilla or Almond Extract

Bread Pudding

Cut or tear bread into small pieces and place in small ramekin or Microwave safe bowl. Blend egg with milk and extract and pour on bread. Use fork to press down bread to soak up all the liquid. Microwave for 45 seconds or adjust time until custard forms.

Day 16

Breakfast	Grapenuts – ½ cup	
	½ cup Milk	
	1 cup Green Tea or Coffee	
Lunch	4 oz. Salmon	
	Tossed Salad with 1 tbsp. Dressing	
	Pita Bread – ½	
	1 cup Green Tea	
Snack	Fresh Fruit	Around 3 PM
Dinner	Pizza – 2 slices	
	1 cup Green Tea	

Honesty

Be honest with yourself. No one else knows what you are eating, or if you are exercising, but you will know. Remember you are doing this for yourself. You deserve to look good in your clothes and to be healthy.

Day 17

Breakfast	Oatmeal Weight Control 1 cup Green Tea or Coffee
Lunch	4 oz. Tuna Pita Bread – ½ Tossed Salad with 1 tbsp. Dressing 1 cup Green Tea
Snack	Fresh Fruit Around 3 PM
Dinner	4 oz. Flounder Red Beets – ½ small can Tossed Salad with 1 tbsp. Dressing 8 oz. Milk

Temptation

We are all tempted from time to time. Don't give up the battle if you should succumb to temptation. Accept it as a way of life and get back on track. One small slip-up will not do too much harm. Pick yourself up, dust yourself off and get on with your life. Then vow to resist the temptation the next time.

Day 18

Breakfast   Eggs – 2
                   Turkey Bacon – 2 slices
                   1 cup Green Tea or Coffee

Lunch   3–4 oz. Sardines
                   Pita Bread – ½
                   Tossed Salad with 1 tbsp. Dressing
                   1 cup Green Tea

Snack   Fresh Fruit   Around 3 PM

Dinner   Chicken Breast – 4 oz
                   Broccoli – 1 cup
                   Mixed Salad
                   8 oz. Milk

Avoid the Kitchen

Don't spend too much time in the kitchen. Do what you have to do and then get out. Staying in the kitchen puts you too close to temptation. Get the food put away, dishes cleaned up and you're out of there.

Day 19

Breakfast	Oatmeal Weight Control
	Apple Sauce – Sugar Free
	1 cup Green Tea or Coffee
Lunch	Shrimp – 8 large
	Homemade Cocktail Sauce
	1 slice Toast
	Tossed Salad with 1 tbsp. Dressing
	1 cup Green Tea
Snack	Fresh Fruit Around 3 PM
Dinner	Ham – 3 slices
	Crushed Pineapple – ¼ cup
	Shredded LF Cheese – ¼ cup
	Whole Wheat Bread - 2 slices
	1 cup Green Tea

Do One Tip per Week

If you do one tip per week, at the end of this session you will have learned four healthy habits at the end of three months that adds up to 12 healthy habits. GO YOU!

Day 20

Breakfast	Cottage Cheese – 4 oz.
	Banana – ½
	Strawberries – 8–10
	Milk – ¾ cup
	Dash of Extract – Vanilla or Almond

Slice fruit and put all ingredients in a blender and blend until smooth

Lunch	1 cup Lentil Soup
	Raisin Bread – 1 slice
	1 cup Green Tea

Snack	Fresh Fruit	Around 3 PM

Dinner	Chopped meat – ¼ pound
	Whole Wheat bread – 1 slice
	Cheese – Velveeta – 1 slice
	Tomato – 1 slice
	Lettuce – 1 leaf

Shape meat into a patty and broil. Place cooked patty on bread and top with tomato and then slice of cheese. Broil until the cheese melts. Use the lettuce leaf as a top to the sandwich.

Do It Now!!

If you want to make changes, DO IT NOW!! Not tomorrow or Monday or next week. The sooner you start the quicker you will reach your goal.

Day 21

Breakfast   Eggs – 2
                      Turkey Bacon – 2 slices
                      Raisin Bread – 1 slice
                      8 oz. Milk

Lunch   3–4 oz. Sardines
                      Pita Bread – ½
                      Tossed Salad with 1 tbsp. Dressing
                      1 cup Green Tea

Snack   Fresh Fruit   Around 3 PM

Dinner   TV Dinner
                      Mixed Salad
                      8 oz. Milk

Love Yourself

You are a wonderful, unique person. You deserve to look good and be healthy. Don't wait another day to implement the changes you need to make to achieve your goal.

Fourth Week

Weigh yourself first thing in the morning and take your measurements, chest, waist, hips and thighs.

Day 22

Breakfast   Grapenuts – ½ cup
4 oz. Milk
1 cup Green Tea or Coffee

Lunch   3–4 oz. Sardines
Pita Bread – ½
Tossed Salad with 1 tbsp. Dressing
1 cup Green Tea

Snack   Fresh Fruit   Around 3 PM

Dinner   Turkey slices – 3-4
Crushed Pineapple – ¼ cup
Shredded LF Cheese – ¼ cup
Whole Wheat Bread - 2 slices
1 cup Green Tea

Prepare the same as with the Ham slices

Obesity

Health problem risks are greatly elevated. The extra weight can cause physical problems like bone and joint problems. And things like diabetes, heart disease, cancers and other serious conditions are more likely to occur.

Day 23

Breakfast	Eggs – 2
	Turkey Bacon – 2 slices
	1 slice Toast
	1 cup Green Tea or Coffee
Lunch	Peanut Butter – 1 tbsp.
	Raisin Bread – 1 slice
	8 oz. Milk
Snack	Fresh Fruit Around 3 PM
Dinner	Chopped meat – ¼ pound
	Whole Wheat bread – 1 slice
	Cheese – Velveeta – 1 slice
	Tomato – 1 slice
	Lettuce – 1 leaf

Shape meat into a patty and broil. Place cooked patty on bread and top with tomato and then slice of cheese. Broil until the cheese melts. Use the lettuce leaf as a top to the sandwich.

Wait 20 Minutes

Wait 20 minutes after eating. If you still feel hungry (which I doubt) then have a piece of fruit.

Day 24

Breakfast	Oatmeal Weight Control
	Applesauce Sugar Free
	1 cup Green Tea or Coffee
Lunch	4 oz. Tuna
	Tossed Salad with 1 tbsp. Dressing
	Pita Bread – ½
	1 cup Green Tea
Snack	Fresh Fruit Around 3 PM
Dinner	TV Dinner
	Tossed Salad
	8 oz. Milk

Brush Your Teeth

Brush your teeth right after your dinner meal. With your teeth fresh and clean you are reluctant to get them dirty. Hence you will resist nibbling in front of the TV.

Day 25

Breakfast   Cottage Cheese – 4 oz.
Banana – ½
Strawberries 8–10
Milk – ¾ cup
Dash of Extract – Vanilla or Almond

Slice fruit and place all ingredients in blender and blend until smooth

Lunch   3-4 oz. Sardines
Pita Bread – ½
Tossed Salad with 1 tbsp. Dressing
1 cup Green Tea

Snack   Fresh Fruit   Around 3 PM

Dinner   TV Dinner
Tossed Salad
8 oz. Milk

Feeling Full

Going to a party? Wear an outfit with a belt and pull the belt tight. As you are eating, when you start to feel full, don't loosen the belt but instead, STOP EATING. You would be surprised at how well this works.

Day 26

Breakfast	Pancakes – 4
	1 tsp. Jelly
	1 cup Green Tea or Coffee
Lunch	4 oz. Salmon
	Pita Bread – ½
	Tossed Salad with 1 tbsp. Dressing
	1 cup Green Tea
Snack	Fresh Fruit Around 3 PM
Dinner	4 oz. Chicken Breast
	1 cup Broccoli
	Mixed Salad
	8 oz. Milk

9-Inch Dinner Plate

Measure the size of the dinner plate you are using. Is it 12 inches? That's too large. Look among your china and find a plate that is 9 inches or less. Or buy paper plates that are smaller, try the luncheon plates. The less room you have on your plate, the less food you can pile on it.

Day 27

Breakfast   Cottage Cheese – 4 oz.
Banana ½
Strawberries – 8-10
Milk – ¾ cup
Dash of Extract – Vanilla or Almond

Slice fruit and place all of the ingredients
into a blender and blend until smooth

Lunch   Peanut Butter – 1 tbsp.
Raisin Bread – 1 slice
8 oz. Milk

Snack   Fresh Fruit   Around 3 PM

Dinner   4 oz. Flounder
Red Beets – ½ small can
Tossed Salad with 1 tbsp. Dressing
1 cup Green Tea

Watching TV

During the commercials do some exercise such as push-ups, sit-ups, squats or walking in place? Whatever you like to do, but do something other than sitting on the couch and vegetating.

Day 28

Breakfast	Eggs – 2
	Turkey Bacon – 2 slices
	Toast – 1 slice
	1 cup Green Tea or Coffee
Lunch	Beef Barley Soup – 1 cup
	Whole Wheat Toast – 1 slice
	1 cup Green Tea
Snack	Fresh Fruit Around 3 PM
Dinner	Have dinner out to celebrate
	You deserve it after all your hard work

BMI

BMI – Metabolic and weight loss calculator
Go to this or any website to check your BMI.

http://health.msn.com/weight-loss/bmi-calculator.aspx

Has your BMI gone down? That's great and will add years to your life. If not, try harder next time. You can do this.

In Closing

If you need to lose more weight, repeat from Day 1 to Day 28 or reverse and go from Day 28 to Day 1. Another way is to pick and choose the days you want to repeat. You can also swap Lunches around or Breakfasts, etc. The possibilities are endless. Be creative, it's fun.

Bonus Week

Normal Eating Menus

Day 1

Breakfast Eggs – 2
Turkey Bacon – 2 slices
1 cup Green Tea or Coffee

Lunch Chopped Meat – 1.4 pound (93% Lean)
Hamburger Roll – 1
Lettuce Leaf – 1
Tomato – 1 slice
Ketchup – 1 tbsp.

Snack Fresh Fruit

Dinner 3 oz. Poached Salmon
Sweet Potato – 1 small
Tossed Salad with Cucumbers
8 oz. Milk

Comments:

Day 2

Breakfast	Cottage Cheese – 4 oz. Toast – 1 slice Strawberry Jelly – ½ tbsp. 1 cup Green Tea or Coffee
Lunch	French toast – 2 slices 1 cup Green Tea or Coffee
Snack	Fresh Fruit
Dinner	Baked Chicken Breast – 3 oz. Baked Potato – ½ small Butter – 1 pat Broccoli – 1 cup Sherbet – 1/2 cup

Comments:

Day 3

Breakfast	Cottage Cheese – 4 oz.
	Banana – ½
	Strawberries – 8 – 10
	Milk – ¾ cup
	Extract
Lunch	Cheese Blintz – 2
	2 tbsp. Sour Cream
	1 cup Green Tea or Coffee
Snack	Fresh Fruit
Dinner	3 oz. Calves Liver
	Onion – 1 – sliced thin
	Red Beets – ½ small can
	8 oz. Milk

Comments:

Day 4

Breakfast	Oatmeal
	Applesauce – Sugar free
	1 cup Green Tea or Coffee

Lunch   Ham – Pineapple – Cheese Sandwich
                      8 oz. Milk

Snack   Fresh Fruit

Dinner   Lamb Chops – 4 oz.
                      Sweet Potato – 1 small
                      Tossed Salad with Cucumbers
                      8 oz. Milk

Comments:

Day 5

Breakfast   Pancakes – 4 small
Strawberry Jelly – ½ tbsp.
1 cup Green Tea or Coffee

Lunch   Crab Meat – ¼ cup
Toast – 2 slices
1 tbsp. Mayonnaise
Lettuce Leaf – 1
Tomato – 1 slice
1 cup Green Tea

Snack   Fresh Fruit

Dinner   3 oz. BBQ Ribs
Baked Potato – ½ small
Butter – 1 pat
Frozen Mixed Vegetables – 1 cup
Sherbet – ½ cup

Comments:

Day 6

Breakfast   Grapenuts – ½ cup
4 oz. Milk
1 cup Green Tea or Coffee

Lunch   3-4 oz. Sardines
Pita Bread – ½
Tossed Salad with 1 tbsp. Dressing
1 cup Green Tea

Snack   Fresh Fruit

Dinner   4 oz. Stuffed Flounder
Sweet Potato – 1 small
Tossed Salad with 1 tbsp. Dressing
8 oz. Milk

Comments:

Day 7

Breakfast	Cottage Cheese – 4 oz.
	Banana – ½
	Blueberries – ½ cup
	Milk – ¾ cup
	Dash of Extract
Lunch	Shrimp – 12 large
	Cocktail Sauce (Homemade)
	Broccoli – 1 cup
	1 cup Green Tea
Snack	Fresh Fruit
Dinner	Filet Mignon – Lean, broiled
	Sweet Potato – 1 small
	Frozen – Mixed Vegetables – 1 cup
	8 oz. Milk

Comments:

Great Tips on Losing Weight

Everyone you talk to seems to have dozens of tips on losing weight. Some are good common sense tips, but some seem to come out of left field. Even people, who can't seem to successfully lose weight and keep it off, seem happy to offer up tips and advice to other people. That's a pretty good indication that many of us know the best advice and tips on losing weight, but we just don't follow them very well. Here are some tips, which, if you use them in your daily journey toward losing weight, can help you.

Use smaller plates. This is one of those tips on losing weight that often makes people roll their eyes. It has nothing to do with eating or exercise, but it really does trick your mind into thinking you're eating more food. A smaller plate will look fuller than a large plate if they have the same amount of food on them. You might even naturally put less food on the smaller plate, to keep it from looking so loaded down. It's a mental trick, but you should try it because it works for many people.

Eat slowly. This is one of the oldest and most popular tips on losing weight. Have you ever watched a speed-eating contest? Imagine someone eating the same amount of food as the winner, but imagine him or her eating it slowly. The champion may have eaten 20 pies in very little time. Could you actually sit down with a fork and slowly eat 20 pies? It's not likely.

The speed eater ate so fast; his body didn't even have time to scream, "STOP, I'M FULL!" And if it had, he was only focused on putting more and more food in, just as we are when we're "starving" and we gulp down our food. Eat slowly and you'll reach a pleasant feeling of fullness rather than the one that means you've eaten too much too fast.

Watch your portion sizes. If fried chicken is your favorite, you might start out with 2 or 3 pieces on your plate. Try grabbing one small piece instead, and filling up on salad or green veggies to replace those missing pieces of chicken. Try to keep a portion of food about the size of your fist. Those mashed potatoes that you don't want to give up? Still eat them, but stop after one small portion, instead of piling a mountain on your plate.

Ten Foods That Speed Metabolism

Are you looking for foods that speed metabolism? This will probably surprise you. All foods speed metabolism.

"How is that possible?" you ask.

Let's take a quick look at just what is metabolism and how does it work. This explanation might help you to better understand the process and how it can affect your body.

When you eat a meal, your body begins the process of digesting the food, drawing out the nutrients and processing them to create energy that keeps your body functioning properly and effectively. It takes approximately 4 hours just to absorb the nutrients. This is repeated with every meal you eat. In a day, that amounts to 12 hours that your body is busy absorbing each meal's nutrients.

In short, during the digestion process, our bodies burn calories. This is especially true of foods containing carbohydrates and protein, which take longer than other foods to digest. Simply by eating, digesting and absorbing nutrients from the food, you speed your metabolism.

Does this mean you should eat more to constantly stimulate calorie burning?

Here's another answer that might surprise you. Yes. But hold on before you park yourself in front of the refrigerator, bib in place, knife and fork at the ready.

If you skip breakfast and other meals, you will reduce how quickly your body burns calories. In this case, eating more food will help speed metabolism. In fact, by eating smaller meals more often throughout the day, you can keep your metabolism working so that your body is constantly in the state of calorie burning.

As mentioned, there are some foods that require more of your body's energy to burn. The degree to which they affect your body's metabolism depends on the particular food choice. Caffeine, coffee, tea, chocolate and a chemical found in chilies are some foods that speed metabolism, but only minimally.

Carbohydrates and protein trigger the highest rate of metabolism. In fact, a protein meal can burn as much as 25% of that meal's calories through digestion and absorption.

While a high protein meal might sound appealing, consider that it would not provide your body with its required round of nutrients. Adding vitamin and mineral supplements is not the answer either, because they do not provide the same quality of nutrients that are found naturally in foods.

Your best choice is to eat well-balanced meals regularly that contain protein, non-starchy vegetables, fats and carbohydrates. This can minimize fat production while keeping your blood sugar at a level that helps to burn fat and build muscle.

Focus on these 10 specific foods that help speed metabolism and burn fat.

Whole grain bread
Chicken
Salmon
Eggs
Fresh Cheese
Green Beans
Summer Squash
Cabbage
Asparagus and other non-starchy vegetables
And, of course, protein rich meats

To temporarily boost your metabolism by as much as 30%, drink cold water.

Remember, there are other factors beyond your control that can affect your body's speed of metabolism, including your age, sex and any medical conditions.

Weight Loss Plan For Teens

Here is a weight loss plan for teens that any parent can also enjoy and experience:

WEEKEND EXERCISES

Schedule weekend activities with your kids that will promote physical exercises. Try activities like biking; wall climbing, a ball game, or swimming. These will be good for your kid and great for your health too!

EATING HEALTHY

You must learn to encourage your kids to eat healthier. A lot of kids nowadays would prefer a trip to a fast food joint than eating vegetables or fruits. Learn to be creative in preparing vegetables as part of the family meal. Experiment on vegetable recipes and encourage your teenager to help you with the preparation, while doing this, talk about the benefits of vegetables and fruits. You may talk about how a certain vegetable can make their skin healthier and avoid common skin problems during puberty. Prepare their lunch when they need to eat in school. You will be surprised at how unhealthy and gross the school canteens are. Make sure to send him to school with a healthy packed lunch.

ENCOURAGE SPORTS

Now, not all teenagers are into sports. But sport is a good way to train kids to become team players and leaders. It is also a very effective factor that can help your weight loss plan for teens. Introduce them to simple sports and find out which interests them. It is important to note though that sports should not be imposed to disguise your weight loss plans for teens in your family. Introduce sports activities to them and see which sports they have interest in and start from there. If your teenager is not into sports, you may want to shift to a different activity that would still encourage them to get some form of exercise. For example, a teenager who has interests in books may not want to engage in a ball game. Make a sport out of it by engaging your teenager to a game of who can walk to the bookstore faster.

Peanut Butter Diet

If you are one of those millions of overweight Americans, you may have heard of the Amazing Peanut Butter Diet, but are you sure about where this diet came from? Are you skeptical about its ability to really help people lose weight? Isn't peanut butter high in fat? Is it really healthy to focus on one particular type of "miracle food" when dieting? These are the types of questions that should be addressed when contemplating any diet, but especially the Amazing Peanut Butter Diet.

It is certainly true that Americans love Peanut Butter; whether it is the fancy kinds you get from little gourmet shops that tout their "all-natural" goodness or the mass-produced kinds that we all grew up with. So let's address some of the above questions about the Amazing Peanut Butter Diet.

First of all, the Amazing Peanut Butter Diet was introduced to America via "Prevention" magazine. It was so popular, the publishers of the magazine created a whole book about it, which you can order from Amazon or pick up off the shelf at your local bookstore. "Prevention" has a good reputation, and as a result, the Amazing Peanut Butter Diet has a good reputation, as well.

So, the first question is answered and now we need to address the second. Can the Amazing Peanut Butter Diet really help people lose weight? Well, believe it or not, there are some studies that show that the Amazing Peanut Butter Diet did actually help people lose weight.

A control-group study was done in Boston; half the overweight participants were given a low-fat diet. The other half were given about 35% of their total calories as

47

monounsaturated fats – the kind found in Peanut Butter, olive oil, and the like. Everything else remained the same – i.e., both groups ate the same number of calories.

For women, the number of calories was 1200 per day. So, what happened? Both groups lost about the same amount of weight, but the upside (for Peanut Butter lovers and peanut farmers) is that the folks who got to eat the creamy goodness stuck to their diet better than the other half of participants did. Although this seems like quite good news at first glance, it is probably important to realize that 1200 calories is hardly any calories. Just about any woman who only eats 1200 calories per day is going to lose weight.

Looking for a dependable way to lose weight fast?

Stop wasting your time with the latest fad diets and miracle pills. The only proven method for weight loss is to eat better and exercise more. You will see better results by gradually making these adjustments as part of an overall healthier lifestyle instead of as a temporary crash diet. This article will suggest a few nutritious foods you can eat that will also fill you up.

Potatoes are one of the healthiest vegetables out there, but they often get a bad reputation as a fatty food because of their high Carb content. The truth is, carbohydrates are not bad themselves, and the problem is when processed carbohydrates make up a large part of a person's daily intake. Starchy carbohydrates such as the ones in potatoes are actually beneficial to the body and should be a part of your every day diet. An average sized potato by itself only has around 100 calories, yet will make you feel full if topped with the right low-fat condiments.

The mistake most people make when adding potatoes into their diet is to top them with all sorts of fatty foods. Butter, sour cream, bacon, and cheese may make for a great loaded baked potato, but they also add a ton of fat and calories to an otherwise healthy meal. Substitute low-fat cheese, nonfat yogurt, and low fat margarine to keep that same delicious taste without sacrificing your diet. Leave the peel on the potato for extra fiber and nutrition.

Fruits and vegetables are an important part of a healthy diet. In addition to providing plenty of nutrients and fiber themselves, they are an easy way to prevent you from choosing an unhealthy alternative. Reaching for an apple instead of a bag of chips will remove a lot of calories, fat, and sodium from your daily intake. To lose weight fast, you should aim to get most of your calories from fruits and vegetables instead of fat and processed carbohydrates.

Free Calorie Counters On Line

There are a number of free calorie counters available on the Internet. These programs allow you to select a specific food and it will tell you how many calories are in one serving. It will also tell you what the recommended serving size is. If you are on a diet, you owe it to yourself to check out the free calorie counters out there.

What should you look for in a calorie counter and how will you know when you have found a good one? This article looks at the basic components of free calorie counters and shows you some of the sophisticated options out there.

Free calorie counters should include basic groceries. An apple is an apple is an apple, no matter how you slice it. Included in this category are dairy, eggs, fruit, meat, poultry, seafood, and vegetables.

But, so much of what we eat today is processed food. So, a good program will also include various branded foods. For instance, you should be able to find out that one serving of Jif Extra Crunchy Peanut Butter equals 2 tablespoons and has 190 calories in it. Additionally, you might find that 16 percent of the food comes from protein, 71 percent from fat, and 14 from Carbs. It has 2 grams of fiber.

Additionally, many free calorie counters include the foods from popular restaurants and fast food outlets. You might be surprised at just how many calories some of your favorite restaurant foods have in them. And, you should take note that most of the time you will consume fewer calories if you go to a hamburger shop than a sit down restaurant.

The calorie counters depend on your ability to judge a serving. Too many times what we judge to be enough for a meal is really multiple servings. To help you with this, the free calorie counters divide foods into their standard suggested serving sizes and tell you what the weight in grams for that amount is.

While most programs simply list the calories in foods, some free calorie counters have a companion program that shows you just how many calories you've burned by doing specific activities.

Everyone knows that the way you lose weight is to burn more calories than you consume in a given period. To lose 1 pound, you must burn 3500 extra calories than you eat.

Detoxification For Your Body

Detoxification is not just for the movie stars who abuse painkillers anymore. New evidence has shown that just about everyone needs Detox – not for drug use, but to clean out the colon, blood system, liver, and other organs that have been building up potentially toxic amounts of unhealthy matter over the years. Lots of people are jumping on the Detox diet bandwagon, and for good reason, too.

With all the preservatives, hormones, air pollutants, pesticides, and even fat (think fast food) that gets into our bodies every day, it just makes sense to clean the temple from time to time. You wouldn't go without cleaning the house for very long, and you shouldn't go very long without cleaning out the body, either.

Here are three delicious recipes for Detox diets. Give them a try if you want to help cleanse your system and/or lose some weight:

1) Veggie Broth

- A head of fresh broccoli
- A cup of fresh spinach leaves
- A stalk of celery
- A pot full of distilled water

Simply cut up the vegetables into very small pieces. Put them in the pot of water, cover, and bring them to a full boil. Then, reduce the heat to a simmer and let all those nutrients seep out of the vegetables into the water. After about thirty minutes, drain the mixture. Discard the

51

vegetables, and drink the broth. Yummy and a good colon cleanser!

2) Tomato-based Hearty Detox Soup

- A pot of purified water
- A head of green cabbage
- Two medium green bell peppers (or one large and one small)
- An onion
- Three stalks of celery
- Three carrots
- One-third to one-half of a pound of fresh or frozen green beans
- One or two cans of diced tomatoes or tomato sauce

Slice the cabbage into strips. Chop the peppers into bite-size pieces or smaller if you prefer. Cut up the onion, celery, and carrots into pieces of the same size. Prepare the green beans.

Some folks will say to add the ingredients to the water a little at a time, beginning with the "hardest" vegetables first. I find that unnecessary. Just throw all the vegetables into the pot of water, cover, and bring to a boil. Then, lower the heat and allow the soup to simmer for several hours. Enjoy! Try making in your crock-pot.

3) Lemon and Citrus "Tea" Detox Recipes

Lemon is quickly becoming a popular Detox ingredient, probably because of its high citric acid content, vitamin C density, and abundance of bioflavonoid. Besides for all these benefits, there is something that is generally pleasing about the lemon, don't you think? Lemon furniture polish still brings back childhood memories of helping my mom dust the living room furniture, my dishwashing detergent is lemon-scented, and lemonade on a hot day – are you kidding? It gets no better than that.

- A glass of grapefruit juice
- The juice of one large lemon
- Two teaspoons of olive oil
- One to two teaspoons of flaxseed oil
- Optional – a clove of crushed garlic
- Optional – split the juices to half a glass of grapefruit and half glass of orange
- A scoop of your favorite protein powder from the nutrition store

Simply combine the above ingredients in your blender and drink. Try to drink it on an empty stomach; perhaps the first thing in the morning, and be prepared to be cleaned out.

Recipes for Detox diets are a sure and fast way to help clean your digestive system out as a whole. However, it is important for you to follow the directions carefully and only use for the length of time that is appropriate.

Green Tea Health Benefits

Are you one of the hundreds of thousands of people who need to lose weight in order to stay healthy? But you just can't afford to spend $10.00 a day or more on special weight loss packages. How would you like to learn about the inexpensive green tea health benefits and how it can help you lose weight? This article will give you some down to earth tips about green tea and its benefits.

Green tea health benefits are almost a given. But as always when you are about to start a special diet with a supplement of any kind; you should always check with your doctor. When you do this you will know you are not endangering your health.

A great many people who are overweight are prone to developing high blood pressure and other related cardiovascular diseases. If you fall into this category you may not be able to use other diet supplements due to the increased danger of kicking your heart rate up higher. However, green tea will not increase your heart rate.

Recent studies have shown that green tea can help you lose weight by increasing your energy levels and speed up the conversion of fat into energy. As you gain this increase in your energy levels you will be able to safely step up your exercise program. The increased exercise will stimulate your metabolic rate, which in turn will burn your calorie intake more efficiently.

One of the ingredients found in green tea is called catechin. A good number of scientists have theorized the large amount of catechin is what enables the green tea to have a dramatic impact on your energy levels. Some believe it increases the output of energy by as much as four percent.

Another of the green tea health benefits is its amazing ability to help the body eliminate toxic body waste. When it acts as an antioxidant it is believed it helps improve your body's immune system. And the end result of this action is you have less chance of becoming ill.

One thing you will notice with the green tea is the quick burning of calories. This may tend to increase your craving for certain foods to replace the calories you have already burned. It's important for you to remember to control your calorie intake. If you should increase the calorie intake you are decreasing the chances of you losing any weight.

Green tea and a controlled calorie intake should allow you to have a gradual loss of weight over an extended period of time. However, if you should want to increase the weight loss more quickly, you reduce your calorie intake even further. In the mean while you would want to increase the amount of exercise, which will also, help speed up the weight loss.

There is one little drawback to green tea. You may be put off by the taste, however as you continue to drink it you will get used to it. If you just can't stomach it you can always try the green tea extract.

By sticking with your controlled diet, exercise and the green tea, you stand an excellent chance of losing all those extra pounds and keeping them off. Clearly the green tea health benefits far out weigh the one little drawback of a different taste.